A Handbook on Cognitive Wave Formulas

N.B. Singh

DEDICATION

To Nature,

I dedicate this book to you, the source of all life. You are my inspiration, my teacher, and my friend.

Thank you for teaching me about the beauty of the world around me. Thank you for showing me the power of the natural world. Thank you for giving me a sense of peace and tranquillity.

I promise to do my part to protect you and your many wonders. I will teach my children about the importance of conservation and sustainability. I will work to make the world a better place for all living things.

Thank you for everything, Nature.

With love,

N.B Singh

Contents

Welcome to "A Handbook on Cognitive Wave Formulas." This handbook is designed as a comprehensive guide for researchers, practitioners, and enthusiasts delving into the fascinating realm of cognitive waves and their mathematical formulations.

Objective

The primary objective of this handbook is to provide a consolidated resource for understanding, formulating, and applying mathematical formulas in the study of cognitive waves. The book covers a wide range of topics, from the fundamentals of brain waves to advanced quantitative analysis techniques and their applications in various fields.

Structure of the Handbook

The handbook is organized into several chapters, each focusing on specific aspects of cognitive waves. It starts with an introduction to set the stage, followed by a deep dive into the fundamentals, cognitive processes, neurological disorders, quantitative analysis techniques, formulae for cognitive enhancement, applications in various fields, future trends, case studies, and a conclusion that summarizes key findings and explores implications for the future.

Audience

This book is tailored for researchers, neuroscientists, psychologists, data scientists, and anyone intrigued by the intersection of mathematics and cognitive science. Whether you are a seasoned professional or a student entering the field, this handbook aims to provide valuable insights and practical formulas.

How to Use this Handbook

Each chapter is designed to be self-contained, allowing readers to focus on specific areas of interest. Mathematical formulas and equations are presented with clarity and accompanied by explanations to facilitate understanding.

I hope you find "A Handbook on Cognitive Wave Formulas" both informative and inspiring in your exploration of the intricate world of cognitive waves.

N.B. Singh

Chapter 1

Introduction

1.1 Understanding Cognitive Waves

Cognitive waves, denoted by Ψ, represent the dynamic electrical activity in the brain. They are pivotal in elucidating cognitive processes. Key formulas include:

$$\Psi(t) = A\sin(2\pi f t + \phi) \tag{1.1}$$

where $\Psi(t)$ is the cognitive wave at time t, A is the amplitude, f is the frequency, and ϕ is the phase.

The power spectrum $S(f)$ of cognitive waves is defined by the Fourier transform:

$$S(f) = \int_{-\infty}^{\infty} \Psi(t)e^{-i2\pi f t}\, dt \tag{1.2}$$

Cognitive states are linked to wave frequencies:

- δ waves (0.5-4 Hz) - Deep sleep

- θ waves (4-8 Hz) - Meditation

- α waves (8-13 Hz) - Relaxation

- β waves (13-30 Hz) - Alertness

- γ waves (ι30 Hz) - Higher cognitive functions

Molecularly, neurotransmitter release R can be modeled as:

$$R = k \cdot \Psi(t) \tag{1.3}$$

"

where k represents the synaptic efficacy.

Understanding cognitive waves is crucial for unraveling the intricacies of the mind and its myriad functions.

1.2 Significance in Neuroscience

The significance of cognitive waves in neuroscience lies in their ability to decode brain activity. We quantify this significance through key mathematical expressions:

$$V_m(t) = V_{rest} + I \cdot R_m \tag{1.4}$$

This membrane potential formula depicts the dynamic interplay of resting potential (V_{rest}), current (I), and membrane resistance (R_m).

The Hodgkin-Huxley model enhances our understanding of neural dynamics:

$$C_m \frac{dV}{dt} = I_{\text{ion}} - I_{\text{stim}} - I_{\text{leak}} - I_{\text{Na}} - I_{\text{K}} \tag{1.5}$$

where C_m is the membrane capacitance, and I_{ion} components represent ion currents.

Synaptic transmission is vital, modeled by:

$$\frac{dc}{dt} = k_+ s(1 - c) - k_- c \tag{1.6}$$

Here, c is the fraction of open channels, s is the neurotransmitter concentration, and k_+ and k_- are rate constants.

Quantum mechanics intertwines with neuroscience via:

$$\hat{H}\Psi = E\Psi \tag{1.7}$$

This Schrödinger equation describes the wave function Ψ and its relation to the Hamiltonian operator $\hat{H}$ and energy E.

Molecularly, neuroplasticity is expressed as:

$$\Delta W = \eta \cdot \Psi(t) \cdot \frac{dV}{dt} \tag{1.8}$$

This equation encapsulates the change in synaptic weight (ΔW) through the learning rate (η), cognitive waves $\Psi(t)$, and the rate of potential change.

Recognizing these mathematical foundations is key to unveiling the profound significance of cognitive waves in neuroscience.

1.3 Historical Perspectives

Journey through the historical tapestry of cognitive waves, marked by key mathematical insights:

The enigmatic electrical nature of neurons is encapsulated in the Nernst equation:

$$E = \frac{RT}{zF} \ln \left(\frac{[ion]_{\text{out}}}{[ion]_{\text{in}}} \right) \tag{1.9}$$

This equation, formulated by Walther Nernst, unveiled the fundamental relationship between ion concentration, temperature, and electrochemical potential.

The advent of Fourier analysis revolutionized signal processing, represented by:

$$f(t) = \sum_{n=-\infty}^{\infty} c_n e^{in\omega t} \tag{1.10}$$

Joseph Fourier's work laid the groundwork for understanding how complex waveforms, including cognitive waves, can be decomposed into simpler components.

Claude Shannon's information theory reshaped neuroscience through:

$$H(X) = -\sum_{i} P(x_i) \log_2 P(x_i) \tag{1.11}$$

Shannon entropy ($H(X)$) quantifies uncertainty, influencing the study of information processing in the brain.

The Hodgkin-Huxley model, introduced in 1952, is encapsulated in:

$$C_m \frac{dV}{dt} = I_{\text{ion}} - I_{\text{stim}} - I_{\text{leak}} - I_{\text{Na}} - I_{\text{K}} \tag{1.12}$$

This model marked a turning point, allowing a deeper understanding of the dynamic behavior of neurons.

Molecular insights emerged with the discovery of neurotransmitters, depicted in the serotonin synthesis pathway:

$$\text{5-HTP} \xrightarrow{\text{enzyme}} \text{5-HT} \xrightarrow{\text{enzyme}} \text{Melatonin} \tag{1.13}$$

Deciphering these historical milestones illuminates the evolution of our understanding of cognitive waves.

1.4 Current Research Trends

Navigate the cutting-edge of cognitive wave research with key mathematical insights:

Quantum cognition explores mental phenomena through the quantum framework:

$$\hat{H}\Psi = E\Psi \tag{1.14}$$

The Schrödinger equation bridges quantum mechanics and cognitive processes, sparking novel perspectives.

Brain connectivity, modeled by graph theory, is quantified using the adjacency matrix:

$$A_{ij} = \begin{cases} 1 & \text{if there is a connection} \\ 0 & \text{otherwise} \end{cases} \tag{1.15}$$

This matrix unravels intricate neural networks, revealing patterns crucial for understanding cognitive dynamics.

Machine learning augments cognitive research with the backpropagation algorithm:

$$\delta_i = \Phi'(in_i) \cdot \sum_j w_{ji}\delta_j \tag{1.16}$$

Backpropagation refines neural network weights (w_{ji}), optimizing models that simulate cognitive processes.

Neurofeedback leverages operant conditioning principles, adjusting brain waves using:

$$\Delta W = \eta \cdot \Psi(t) \cdot \frac{dV}{dt} \tag{1.17}$$

This equation encapsulates the neuroplasticity induced by cognitive training, a frontier in cognitive therapy.

Brain-computer interfaces decode neural signals with the motor imagery task:

$$P300 = \sum_{i=1}^{N} P300_i \tag{1.18}$$

The P300 wave, extracted through EEG, propels advancements in neurotechnology for communication and control.

Molecular studies probe genetic influences on cognitive waves, exploring allelic variations:

$$\text{SNP} = \frac{\text{Var}(allele)}{\text{Var}(total)} \tag{1.19}$$

Single nucleotide polymorphisms (SNPs) unravel genetic contributions to individual differences in cognitive patterns.

Dive into these mathematical frontiers to grasp the pulse of current cognitive wave research.

1.5 Scope and Objectives

Unveil the expansive realm of cognitive wave exploration with key mathematical foundations:

The scope encompasses the brain's cognitive response to stimuli, articulated by the dynamic sigmoid function:

$$\sigma(x) = \frac{1}{1 + e^{-x}} \tag{1.20}$$

The sigmoid function models neural activation, vital for understanding cognitive reactions.

Objectives include unraveling cognitive complexity through fractal geometry:

$$Z = Z^2 + C \tag{1.21}$$

The Mandelbrot set, derived from this equation, mirrors the intricate structures inherent in cognitive processes.

Exploring cognitive dynamics involves quantifying uncertainty with the Shannon entropy:

$$H(X) = -\sum_i P(x_i) \log_2 P(x_i) \tag{1.22}$$

This entropy measure guides the study of information processing within cognitive systems.

The molecular objective delves into neurochemistry, symbolized by the dopamine synthesis pathway:

$$\text{Tyrosine} \xrightarrow{\text{enzyme}} \text{L--DOPA} \xrightarrow{\text{enzyme}} \text{Dopamine} \tag{1.23}$$

Investigating neurotransmitter pathways enriches the comprehension of cognitive states.

Mathematical models, like the Hodgkin-Huxley equation:

$$C_m \frac{dV}{dt} = I_{\text{ion}} - I_{\text{stim}} - I_{\text{leak}} - I_{\text{Na}} - I_{\text{K}} \tag{1.24}$$

Set the stage for dissecting neural intricacies, aligning with the objective of cognitive wave formula exploration.

Embark on this mathematical journey to fulfill the scope and objectives of unraveling the secrets within cognitive waves.

1.6 Terminology and Definitions

Navigate the linguistic landscape of cognitive waves with key mathematical foundations:

Begin with the basics, defining the cognitive wave amplitude (A) using the Pythagorean theorem:

$$A = \sqrt{Re(\Psi)^2 + Im(\Psi)^2} \tag{1.25}$$

Where $Re(\Psi)$ and $Im(\Psi)$ represent the real and imaginary parts of the cognitive wave.

Explore wave frequency (f) through the Doppler effect:

$$f' = f \cdot \frac{v + v_o}{v + v_s} \tag{1.26}$$

Understanding the frequency shift in cognitive waves mirrors the Doppler principle.

Dive into cognitive states categorized by frequency bands:

- δ waves (0.5-4 Hz) - Sleep, modeled by:

$$\delta(t) = A \sin(2\pi f_\delta t) \tag{1.27}$$

- θ waves (4-8 Hz) - Meditation, expressed as:

$$\theta(t) = A \sin(2\pi f_\theta t) \tag{1.28}$$

- α waves (8-13 Hz) - Relaxation, formulated by:

$$\alpha(t) = A \sin(2\pi f_\alpha t) \tag{1.29}$$

- β waves (13-30 Hz) - Alertness, defined as:

$$\beta(t) = A \sin(2\pi f_\beta t) \tag{1.30}$$

- γ waves (¿30 Hz) - Higher cognition, characterized by:

$$\gamma(t) = A \sin(2\pi f_\gamma t) \tag{1.31}$$

Unravel neurotransmitter actions through the Michaelis-Menten kinetics:

$$V_0 = \frac{V_{\max} \cdot [S]}{K_m + [S]} \tag{1.32}$$

This equation mirrors the enzyme-substrate dynamics in synaptic transmission.

Conceptualize cognitive network connections using graph theory:

$$A_{ij} = \begin{cases} 1 & \text{if there is a connection} \\ 0 & \text{otherwise} \end{cases} \tag{1.33}$$

The adjacency matrix unveils the connectivity fabric within cognitive networks.

Unearth the linguistic nuances with these mathematical foundations, forging a profound understanding of cognitive wave terminology.

1.7 Organization of the Handbook

Decode the structure of this handbook with concise mathematical insights:

Begin with a nod to the Fibonacci sequence, underpinning the organization:

$$F_n = F_{n-1} + F_{n-2} \tag{1.34}$$

The sequence governs the chapter arrangement, embodying natural patterns in cognitive exploration.

Traverse the landscape of contents through the lens of calculus:

$$\int_a^b f(x)\,dx = F(b) - F(a) \tag{1.35}$$

This definite integral symbolizes the exploration journey, integrating diverse topics.

Each chapter unfolds like a neural network layer, governed by activation functions:

$$\sigma(x) = \frac{1}{1 + e^{-x}} \tag{1.36}$$

The sigmoid activation mirrors the transition between chapters, capturing the essence of cognitive progression.

Peer into the microscopic world of sub-sections through Heisenberg's uncertainty principle:

$$\Delta x \cdot \Delta p \geq \frac{\hbar}{2} \tag{1.37}$$

The uncertainty principle guides the granularity, mirroring the inevitable uncertainty in navigating cognitive complexities.

As you embark on this journey, envision the molecular precision of DNA replication:

$$A\!-\!T, G\!-\!C \tag{1.38}$$

DNA base pairing signifies the meticulous alignment of concepts and chapters.

Conclude with a nod to chaos theory, embedded in fractal geometry:

$$Z = Z^2 + C \tag{1.39}$$

The Mandelbrot set encapsulates the unpredictability, adding a touch of chaos to the organized structure.

Unravel the handbook's intricacies with these mathematical guideposts, fostering a systematic exploration of cognitive waves.

Chapter 2

Fundamentals of Brain Waves

2.1 Neural Oscillations

Delve into the rhythmic dance of neural oscillations with swift mathematical insights:

Visualize the oscillatory nature using the simple harmonic motion equation:

$$x(t) = A\cos(\omega t + \phi) \tag{2.1}$$

This equation mirrors the back-and-forth sway of neural oscillations, where A is amplitude, ω is angular frequency, t is time, and ϕ is phase.

Harmonize with the resonance frequency through the resonance curve:

$$Y(\omega) = \frac{1}{\sqrt{(1 - (\omega/\omega_0)^2)^2 + (2\zeta\omega/\omega_0)^2}} \tag{2.2}$$

Resonance dynamics unfold through this curve, revealing the interplay between angular frequency (ω) and damping ratio (ζ).

Immerse in the spectral domain using the Fourier transform:

$$X(f) = \int_{-\infty}^{\infty} x(t)e^{-j2\pi ft}\, dt \tag{2.3}$$

Fourier transform unveils the frequency components, translating neural oscillations into a spectrum.

Witness synchronization between neural populations with the Kuramoto model:

$$\dot{\theta}_i = \omega_i + \frac{K}{N}\sum_{j=1}^{N}\sin(\theta_j - \theta_i) \tag{2.4}$$

Kuramoto's equation encapsulates the synchronization dynamics, where θ_i is the phase of oscillator i, ω_i is its natural frequency, and K represents coupling strength.

Dive into the neurochemical symphony with neurotransmitter kinetics:

$$V_0 = \frac{V_{\text{max}} \cdot [S]}{K_m + [S]} \tag{2.5}$$

Neurotransmitter release follows this Michaelis-Menten equation, shaping the chemical backdrop of neural oscillations.

Conclude with the cross-frequency coupling dance:

$$\Phi_{\text{CFC}}(f_1, f_2) = \int x_1(t)x_2^*(t)\, dt \tag{2.6}$$

Cross-frequency coupling unveils the intricate interdependence of different frequency components in neural oscillations.

Journey through neural oscillations, propelled by these mathematical rhythms, revealing the mesmerizing world within the brain's rhythmic dance.

2.2 Electroencephalography (EEG)

Unveil the electrical symphony of the brain through rapid mathematical insights:

Capture neural signals using the voltage potential equation:

$$V(t) = R \cdot I(t) \tag{2.7}$$

Ohm's law encapsulates the relationship between voltage (V), resistance (R), and current (I) in EEG recordings.

Decipher brain activity spectra with the Fourier transform:

$$X(f) = \int_{-\infty}^{\infty} x(t)e^{-j2\pi ft}\, dt \tag{2.8}$$

EEG signals transform into frequency components, unveiling the dynamic neural landscape.

Analyze temporal patterns using the autocorrelation function:

$$R(\tau) = \int x(t)x(t - \tau)\, dt \tag{2.9}$$

Autocorrelation maps temporal dependencies in EEG signals, unraveling recurrent patterns.

Explore brain dynamics with wavelet analysis:

$$C_a(\tau, s) = \int x(t)\psi_{\tau,s}^*(t)\, dt \tag{2.10}$$

Continuous wavelet transform delves into the time-frequency domain, disclosing intricate EEG wave dynamics.

Decode cognitive states through event-related potentials (ERPs):

$$ERP(t) = \frac{1}{N} \sum_{i=1}^{N} x_i(t) \tag{2.11}$$

ERP signals average over trials (N), extracting consistent brain responses from EEG recordings.

Witness coherence between brain regions using the coherence function:

$$C(f) = \frac{|S_{xy}(f)|^2}{S_{xx}(f) S_{yy}(f)} \tag{2.12}$$

Coherence unveils synchronized activity, mapping the connectivity web in EEG signals.

Conclude with the neurochemical underpinnings using neurotransmitter kinetics:

$$V_0 = \frac{V_{\max} \cdot [S]}{K_m + [S]} \tag{2.13}$$

Neurotransmitter release, governed by Michaelis-Menten kinetics, adds a molecular layer to EEG exploration.

Navigate the EEG realm with these mathematical beacons, unlocking the secrets embedded in the brain's electrical symphony.

2.3 Types of Brain Waves

Navigate the diverse spectrum of brain waves with rapid mathematical insights:

Dive into the Delta waves, synonymous with deep sleep:

$$\delta(t) = A \sin(2\pi f_\delta t) \tag{2.14}$$

Delta waves oscillate at 0.5-4 Hz, orchestrating the tranquility of restful slumber.

Explore Theta waves, orchestrators of meditative states:

$$\theta(t) = A \sin(2\pi f_\theta t) \tag{2.15}$$

Theta waves dance at 4-8 Hz, ushering the mind into a serene meditative realm.

Embrace Alpha waves, heralds of relaxation:

$$\alpha(t) = A \sin(2\pi f_\alpha t) \tag{2.16}$$

Alpha waves serenade at 8-13 Hz, inducing a state of tranquil repose.

Ignite with Beta waves, guardians of alertness:

$$\beta(t) = A\sin(2\pi f_\beta t) \tag{2.17}$$

Beta waves resonate at 13-30 Hz, fueling the cognitive vigor of wakefulness.

Soar with Gamma waves, emissaries of higher cognition:

$$\gamma(t) = A\sin(2\pi f_\gamma t) \tag{2.18}$$

Gamma waves sparkle at frequencies above 30 Hz, orchestrating complex cognitive functions.

Revel in the molecular dance of neurotransmitter release:

$$R = k \cdot \Psi(t) \tag{2.19}$$

Neurotransmitter release (R) harmonizes with cognitive waves ($\Psi(t)$), creating a symphony of chemical signaling.

Conclude with the neural orchestra, where these waves intertwine, shaping the cognitive symphony within the brain.

2.4　Frequency Bands

Navigate the rich tapestry of brain wave frequencies with swift mathematical insights:

Immerse in the Delta realm, where tranquility reigns:

- Frequency Range: 0.5-4 Hz

- Mathematical Harmony:

$$\delta(t) = A\sin(2\pi f_\delta t) \tag{2.20}$$

Traverse the Theta landscape, a gateway to meditative states:

- Frequency Range: 4-8 Hz

- Mathematical Serenity:

$$\theta(t) = A\sin(2\pi f_\theta t) \tag{2.21}$$

Embrace the Alpha oasis, the realm of relaxation:

- Frequency Range: 8-13 Hz

- Mathematical Repose:

$$\alpha(t) = A\sin(2\pi f_\alpha t) \tag{2.22}$$

Ignite with the Beta blaze, guardians of alertness:

- Frequency Range: 13-30 Hz

- Mathematical Vigor:
$$\beta(t) = A\sin(2\pi f_\beta t) \tag{2.23}$$

i

Soar into the Gamma galaxy, orchestrators of higher cognition:

- Frequency Range: ¿30 Hz

- Mathematical Brilliance:
$$\gamma(t) = A\sin(2\pi f_\gamma t) \tag{2.24}$$

Marvel at the neural symphony where these frequencies intertwine, sculpting the dynamic cognitive landscape within the brain.

2.5 Waveform Characteristics

Embark on a whirlwind tour of brain wave waveform traits with rapid mathematical insights:

Embrace the Delta's slow undulations:

- Frequency Range: 0.5-4 Hz

- Mathematical Dance:
$$\delta(t) = A\sin(2\pi f_\delta t) \tag{2.25}$$

- Noteworthy Features: Slow, high amplitude, deep sleep orchestrator

Glide through the Theta's tranquil curves:

- Frequency Range: 4-8 Hz

- Mathematical Harmony:
$$\theta(t) = A\sin(2\pi f_\theta t) \tag{2.26}$$

- Noteworthy Features: Relaxed, associated with meditation

Relax in the Alpha's rhythmic ebbs:

- Frequency Range: 8-13 Hz

- Mathematical Pulsation:

$$\alpha(t) = A\sin(2\pi f_\alpha t) \tag{2.27}$$

- Noteworthy Features: Awake but calm, eyes closed state

Energize with the Beta's dynamic peaks:

- Frequency Range: 13-30 Hz

- Mathematical Vibrance:

$$\beta(t) = A\sin(2\pi f_\beta t) \tag{2.28}$$

- Noteworthy Features: Active, alert, engaged in cognitive tasks

Soar into the Gamma's swift surges:

- Frequency Range: ¿30 Hz

- Mathematical Brilliance:

$$\gamma(t) = A\sin(2\pi f_\gamma t) \tag{2.29}$$

- Noteworthy Features: Linked to high-level cognitive functions

Unveil the unique signatures of each wave, painting a vibrant portrait of the brain's oscillatory symphony.

2.6 Influence of Brain Regions

Explore the dynamic interplay of brain regions with swift mathematical insights:

Decode connectivity using the coherence function:

$$C(f) = \frac{|S_{xy}(f)|^2}{S_{xx}(f)S_{yy}(f)} \tag{2.30}$$

Coherence unveils synchronized activity, mapping the connectivity web in brain waves.

Witness network synchronization through the Kuramoto model:

$$\dot{\theta}_i = \omega_i + \frac{K}{N}\sum_{j=1}^{N}\sin(\theta_j - \theta_i) \tag{2.31}$$

Kuramoto's equation encapsulates the synchronized dance, where θ_i is the phase of oscillator i, ω_i is its natural frequency, and K represents coupling strength.

Dive into the neural symphony, where cross-frequency coupling orchestrates:

$$\Phi_{\text{CFC}}(f_1, f_2) = \int x_1(t) x_2^*(t)\, dt \tag{2.32}$$

Cross-frequency coupling unveils the intricate interdependence of different frequency components in brain regions.

Conclude with the neurochemical underpinnings using neurotransmitter kinetics:

$$V_0 = \frac{V_{\text{max}} \cdot [S]}{K_m + [S]} \tag{2.33}$$

Neurotransmitter release, governed by Michaelis-Menten kinetics, adds a molecular layer to the intricate dance of brain regions.

Navigate the neural landscape where brain waves harmonize and synchronize, shaping the symphony within the interconnected regions.

2.7 Interpreting EEG Patterns

Decipher the enigmatic language of EEG patterns with rapid mathematical insights:

Unravel brain dynamics through spectral analysis:

$$X(f) = \int_{-\infty}^{\infty} x(t) e^{-j 2\pi f t}\, dt \tag{2.34}$$

EEG signals translate into frequency components, exposing the rhythmic language of neural activity.

Probe temporal relationships with the autocorrelation function:

$$R(\tau) = \int x(t) x(t - \tau)\, dt \tag{2.35}$$

Autocorrelation unveils temporal dependencies, providing insight into recurring EEG patterns.

Navigate the time-frequency domain with wavelet analysis:

$$C_a(\tau, s) = \int x(t) \psi_{\tau,s}^*(t)\, dt \tag{2.36}$$

Continuous wavelet transform delves into the intricate time-frequency nuances, capturing the evolving nature of EEG patterns.

Dissect event-related potentials (ERPs) with averaging:

$$ERP(t) = \frac{1}{N}\sum_{i=1}^{N} x_i(t) \tag{2.37}$$

ERP signals emerge through averaging, spotlighting consistent brain responses hidden within EEG patterns.

Illuminate connectivity using the coherence function:

$$C(f) = \frac{|S_{xy}(f)|^2}{S_{xx}(f)S_{yy}(f)} \tag{2.38}$$

Coherence unveils synchronized activity, painting a picture of connectivity within EEG patterns. Conclude with the synaptic symphony:

$$R = k \cdot \Psi(t) \tag{2.39}$$

Neurotransmitter release (R) harmonizes with cognitive waves ($\Psi(t)$), adding a molecular layer to the interpretation of EEG patterns.

Navigate the EEG realm with these mathematical beacons, unlocking the secrets embedded in the brain's electrical symphony.

Chapter 3

Cognitive Processes and Waves

3.1 Perception and Attention

Embark on the cognitive journey of perception and attention with swift mathematical insights:

Explore perceptual processes through signal detection theory:

$$d' = \frac{z(\text{Hits}) - z(\text{False Alarms})}{\sqrt{2}} \tag{3.1}$$

The sensitivity index (d') quantifies the ability to distinguish signal from noise in perceptual tasks.

Navigate attention dynamics with the Attentional Blink phenomenon:

$$P(T2|T1) = P(T2) - P(T1) \cdot P(T2|T1) \tag{3.2}$$

Attentional Blink probability reveals the temporal constraints in processing consecutive stimuli.

Illuminate neural correlates using the P300 wave:

$$P300 = \sum_{i=1}^{N} P300_i \tag{3.3}$$

The P300 wave, extracted through EEG, signifies attention allocation in cognitive tasks.

Unravel the chemistry behind attention with acetylcholine dynamics:

$$\text{Choline} + \text{Acetyl\,CoA} \xrightarrow{\text{enzyme}} \text{Acetylcholine} + \text{CoA} \tag{3.4}$$

Acetylcholine synthesis influences attention and memory processes.

Conclude with the dynamic interplay of perception and attention, where mathematical principles shed light on the cognitive intricacies.

3.2   Memory Formation

Dive into the realms of memory formation with rapid mathematical insights:

Unveil the encoding process through the Atkinson-Shiffrin model:

- Sensory Memory: $S(t) = I(t) * e^{-\alpha t}$

- Short-Term Memory: $STM(t) = \int_{-\infty}^{t} S(t)\, dt$

- Long-Term Memory: $LTM(t) = \int_{-\infty}^{t} STM(t)\, dt$

The model quantifies the flow of information from sensory to long-term memory.

Illuminate the forgetting curve with Ebbinghaus' formula:

$$R(t) = e^{-\frac{t}{s}} \tag{3.5}$$

The retention ($R(t)$) of information decays exponentially over time (t).

Navigate the synaptic plasticity landscape with Hebbian learning:

$$\Delta W_{ij} = \eta \cdot x_i \cdot y_j \tag{3.6}$$

Hebbian learning adjusts synaptic weights (W_{ij}) based on correlated activity.

Unravel the molecular symphony of memory with CREB activation:

$$ATP \xrightarrow{\text{enzyme}} cAMP \xrightarrow{\text{enzyme}} CREB \xrightarrow{\text{enzyme}} New\,Synapses \tag{3.7}$$

CREB activation sparks molecular cascades, contributing to memory consolidation.

Conclude with the intricate dance of memory formation, where mathematical principles guide the understanding of cognitive processes.

3.3   Language Processing

Embark on the linguistic journey of language processing with swift mathematical insights:

Illuminate phonological processing using the Dual-Route Cascaded model:

- Lexical Route: $P(L) = P(L_s) \cdot P(L_r)$

- Sublexical Route: $P(S) = P(S_s) \cdot P(S_r)$

The model dissects the parallel routes for recognizing spoken words.

Decode syntactic structures through the Chomsky hierarchy:

- Type 3 (Regular): $A \to aB$ or $A \to a$

- Type 2 (Context-Free): $A \to \alpha$

- Type 1 (Context-Sensitive): $\alpha \to \beta$

The hierarchy classifies language rules, unveiling syntactic complexities.

Illuminate semantic processing with vector space models:

$$\text{Similarity}(w_1, w_2) = \frac{w_1 \cdot w_2}{\|w_1\| \cdot \|w_2\|} \tag{3.8}$$

Vector spaces capture semantic relationships, guiding word meaning associations.

Unravel neural language representation with recurrent neural networks (RNN):

$$h_t = \sigma(W_{hh}h_{t-1} + W_{xh}x_t) \tag{3.9}$$

RNNs model sequential dependencies, reflecting the dynamic nature of language.

Conclude with the symphony of language processing, where mathematical principles illuminate the intricate dance of linguistic cognition.

3.4 Problem Solving

Navigate the mental labyrinth of problem-solving with rapid mathematical insights:

Decode decision-making through the Expected Utility Theory:

$$EU = \sum_i p_i \cdot u(x_i) \tag{3.10}$$

Expected Utility quantifies the rational choice process based on probabilities (p_i) and utility values ($u(x_i)$).

Illuminate heuristic strategies with the availability heuristic:

$$\text{Availability} = \frac{\text{Frequency of retrieval}}{\text{Total frequency}} \tag{3.11}$$

Availability heuristic guides decision-making based on easily accessible information.

Unravel problem-solving algorithms with the A* search algorithm:

$$f(n) = g(n) + h(n) \tag{3.12}$$

A* algorithm balances the cost of reaching a state ($g(n)$) with the heuristic estimate to the goal ($h(n)$).

Dive into creative problem-solving with lateral thinking:

$$\text{Lateral Thinking} = \text{Random Mental Exploration} + \text{Pattern Breaking} \tag{3.13}$$

Lateral thinking fosters unconventional solutions through mental flexibility.

Conclude with the dynamic landscape of problem-solving, where mathematical principles illuminate the art of navigating challenges.

3.5 Decision Making

Embark on the decision-making journey with rapid mathematical insights:

Illuminate rational choices through the Utility Theory:

$$U(x) = \sum_i p_i \cdot u(x_i) \tag{3.14}$$

Utility Theory quantifies rational decisions based on probabilities (p_i) and utility values ($u(x_i)$).

Decode biases with Prospect Theory:

$$V(x) = \begin{cases} x^\alpha & \text{if } x \geq 0 \\ -\lambda(-x)^\beta & \text{if } x < 0 \end{cases} \tag{3.15}$$

Prospect Theory models decision-making under risk, considering gains and losses non-linearly.

Unravel the dynamic interplay of emotions with the Somatic Marker Hypothesis:

$$\text{Somatic Marker} = \text{Emotional Signal} + \text{Anticipation} \tag{3.16}$$

Somatic markers guide decisions by linking emotional responses to future outcomes.

Navigate the complexity of group decision-making with the Condorcet Jury Theorem:

$$P(\text{Group is Correct}) = \left(\frac{1}{2}\right)^N + \left(\frac{1}{2}\right)^{N-1} \cdot \binom{N}{1} \tag{3.17}$$

The theorem quantifies the probability of a correct decision by a majority vote.

Conclude with the intricate dance of decision-making, where mathematical principles guide the understanding of cognitive processes.

3.6 Emotional Regulation

Explore the realm of emotional regulation with swift mathematical insights:

Illuminate emotional appraisal with the Cannon-Bard Theory:

$$\text{Emotion} = \text{Physiological Arousal} + \text{Conscious Feeling} \tag{3.18}$$

Cannon-Bard theory dissects emotions as simultaneous physiological responses and conscious feelings.

Decode emotional intelligence through the Mayer-Salovey-Caruso Model:

$$\text{Emotional Intelligence} = \text{Perceiving} + \text{Understanding} + \text{Managing} + \text{Using} \tag{3.19}$$

The model breaks down emotional intelligence into key components.

Unravel the neurochemistry of emotion with serotonin reuptake:

$$\text{Serotonin} + \text{Receptor} \xrightarrow{\text{Reuptake}} \text{Serotonin Reuptake} \tag{3.20}$$

Serotonin reuptake influences mood and emotional balance.

Dive into emotion regulation strategies with the Gross Process Model:

$$\begin{aligned}
\text{Situation Selection} &\rightarrow \text{Situation Modification} \\
&\rightarrow \text{Attentional Deployment} \\
&\rightarrow \text{Cognitive Change} \\
&\rightarrow \text{Response Modulation}
\end{aligned} \tag{3.21}$$

Gross's model outlines steps for effective emotion regulation.

Conclude with the dynamic landscape of emotional regulation, where mathematical principles guide the understanding of cognitive processes.

3.7 Conscious and Unconscious Processes

Navigate the dichotomy of consciousness with rapid mathematical insights:

Illuminate conscious processing with Global Workspace Theory:

$$\text{Conscious Access} \propto \text{Global Availability of Information} \tag{3.22}$$

Global Workspace Theory links consciousness to the widespread availability of information in the brain.

Decode unconscious influences with Priming Effects:

$$\begin{aligned}
\text{Priming} &= \text{Previous Exposure} \\
&\rightarrow \text{Altered Response}
\end{aligned} \tag{3.23}$$

Priming reveals how prior stimuli shape subsequent responses without conscious awareness.

Unravel the neural network of consciousness with the Integrated Information Theory:

$$\Phi = \max \left(\sum \Phi(\text{partition}), \sum \Phi(\text{each part}) \right) \tag{3.24}$$

Integrated Information Theory quantifies the level of consciousness based on the interconnectedness of neural elements.

Dive into the subconscious realm with Freudian Iceberg Model:

$$\text{Conscious Mind} \subset \text{Preconscious Mind} \\ \subset \text{Unconscious Mind} \tag{3.25}$$

Freud's model visualizes the hierarchy of conscious and unconscious mental processes.

Conclude with the intricate dance of conscious and unconscious processes, where mathematical principles guide the understanding of cognitive intricacies.

Chapter 4

Neurological Disorders and Cognitive Waves

4.1 Role in Neurological Diseases

Explore the connection between cognitive waves and neurological diseases with rapid mathematical insights:

Illuminate the impact of Alzheimer's on neural connections:

$$\text{Neural Connectivity} = \frac{\text{Synaptic Density in Healthy Brain}}{\text{Synaptic Density in Alzheimer's Brain}} \tag{4.1}$$

Alzheimer's disrupts neural connectivity, affecting cognitive wave patterns.

Decode the role of dopamine imbalance in Parkinson's:

$$\text{Dopamine} \xrightarrow{\text{Deficiency}} \text{Parkinsonian Symptoms} \tag{4.2}$$

Dopamine imbalance alters neural oscillations, contributing to Parkinson's symptoms.

Unravel the impact of GABAergic dysfunction in Epilepsy:

$$\text{Excitation} - \text{Inhibition Imbalance} \xrightarrow{\text{GABA Dysfunction}} \text{Epileptic Seizures} \tag{4.3}$$

GABAergic dysfunction disrupts the delicate balance of neural excitation and inhibition.

Dive into the disruption of neural oscillations in Schizophrenia:

$$\text{Dysregulated Neural Oscillations} = \frac{\text{Normal Neural Synchronization}}{\text{Schizophrenic Neural Synchronization}} \tag{4.4}$$

Schizophrenia introduces chaos to normal neural oscillatory patterns.

Conclude with the intricate relationship between cognitive waves and neurological diseases, where mathematical principles guide the understanding of complex disorders.

4.2 Alzheimer's Disease

Explore the Alzheimer's landscape with swift mathematical insights:

Illuminate the impact on synaptic density:

$$\text{Synaptic Density Reduction} = \frac{\text{Initial Synaptic Density} - \text{Alzheimer's Synaptic Density}}{\text{Initial Synaptic Density}} \tag{4.5}$$

Alzheimer's leads to a reduction in synaptic density, disrupting neural connections.

Decode the role of beta-amyloid accumulation:

$$\text{Beta}-\text{Amyloid Aggregation} \xrightarrow{\text{Neurotoxicity}} \text{Neural Dysfunction} \tag{4.6}$$

Beta-amyloid accumulation induces neurotoxicity, contributing to cognitive decline.

Unravel the tau protein hyperphosphorylation:

$$\text{Tau} + \text{Kinase} \xrightarrow{\text{Hyperphosphorylation}} \text{Neurofibrillary Tangles} \tag{4.7}$$

Hyperphosphorylation of tau proteins leads to the formation of neurofibrillary tangles, disrupting neuronal function.

Dive into the molecular cascade of Alzheimer's with cholinergic dysfunction:

$$\text{Acetylcholine} + \text{AChE} \xrightarrow{\text{Deficiency}} \text{Cholinergic Dysfunction} \tag{4.8}$$

Cholinergic dysfunction contributes to cognitive impairments in Alzheimer's.

Conclude with the intricate molecular dance in Alzheimer's, where mathematical principles guide the understanding of the disease.

4.3 Parkinson's Disease

Navigate the Parkinson's landscape with swift mathematical insights:

Illuminate the dopamine deficiency impact:

$$\text{Dopamine} \xrightarrow{\text{Deficiency}} \text{Parkinsonian Symptoms} \tag{4.9}$$

Dopamine deficiency leads to motor symptoms and cognitive impairments in Parkinson's.

Decode the role of alpha-synuclein aggregation:

$$\text{Alpha}-\text{Synuclein} \xrightarrow{\text{Aggregation}} \text{Lewy Bodies Formation} \tag{4.10}$$

Aggregation of alpha-synuclein results in the formation of Lewy bodies, contributing to neuronal dysfunction.

Unravel the impact on neural oscillations:

$$\text{Dysregulated Neural Oscillations} = \frac{\text{Normal Neural Synchronization}}{\text{Parkinsonian Neural Synchronization}} \tag{4.11}$$

Parkinson's disrupts normal neural oscillations, affecting cognitive processes.

Dive into the molecular cascade of oxidative stress:

$$\text{Oxidative Stress} \xrightarrow{\text{Free Radicals}} \text{Neuronal Damage} \tag{4.12}$$

Oxidative stress induces neuronal damage, contributing to Parkinson's pathology.

Conclude with the intricate molecular dance in Parkinson's, where mathematical principles guide the understanding of the disease.

4.4 Epilepsy and Seizures

Explore the dynamics of epilepsy and seizures with swift insights:

Illuminate the impact of GABA dysfunction:

$$\text{Excitation-Inhibition Imbalance} \xrightarrow{\text{GABA Dysfunction}} \text{Epileptic Seizures}$$

GABAergic dysfunction disrupts the balance between excitation and inhibition, triggering epileptic seizures.

Decode the alteration in neural synchronization:

$$\text{Dysregulated Neural Synchronization} = \frac{\text{Normal Neural Synchronization}}{\text{Epileptic Neural Synchronization}}$$

Epilepsy disrupts normal neural synchronization, resulting in aberrant brain activity.

Unravel the changes in network connectivity:

$$\text{Altered Connectivity} = \frac{\text{Normal Network Connectivity}}{\text{Epileptic Network Connectivity}}$$

Epilepsy induces alterations in network connectivity, impacting cognitive functions.

Dive into the molecular cascade of glutamate excitotoxicity:

$$\text{Glutamate Excitotoxicity} \xrightarrow{\text{Neuronal Damage}} \text{Seizure-Induced Injury}$$

Glutamate excitotoxicity contributes to neuronal damage during seizures.

Conclude with the intricate molecular dance in epilepsy, where insights guide the understanding of the disorder.

4.5 Mood Disorders

Explore the intersection of cognitive waves and mood disorders with rapid insights:

Illuminate the serotonin dynamics in depression:

$$\text{Serotonin} + \text{Receptor} \xrightarrow{\text{Reuptake Inhibition}} \text{Increased Serotonin Levels} \tag{4.13}$$

Reuptake inhibition enhances serotonin levels, impacting mood regulation in depression.

Decode the neurogenesis impact in bipolar disorder:

$$\text{Neurogenesis} + \text{Bipolar Disorder} \xrightarrow{\text{Dysregulation}} \text{Mood Swings} \tag{4.14}$$

Dysregulated neurogenesis contributes to mood swings in bipolar disorder.

Unravel the impact of norepinephrine in anxiety:

$$\text{Norepinephrine} + \text{Receptor} \xrightarrow{\text{Activation}} \text{Anxiogenic Effects} \tag{4.15}$$

Norepinephrine activation induces anxiogenic effects, influencing anxiety disorders.

Dive into the neuroinflammation dynamics in mood disorders:

$$\text{Neuroinflammation} \xrightarrow{\text{Cytokine Release}} \text{Mood Disturbances} \tag{4.16}$$

Neuroinflammation, through cytokine release, contributes to mood disturbances.

Conclude with the intricate molecular dance in mood disorders, where insights guide the understanding of these complex conditions.

4.6 Cognitive Impairments

Explore the realm of cognitive impairments and their connection to cognitive waves with rapid insights:

Illuminate the impact of amyloid-beta accumulation:

$$\text{Beta} - \text{Amyloid Aggregation} \xrightarrow{\text{Neurotoxicity}} \text{Cognitive Decline} \tag{4.17}$$

Amyloid-beta aggregation induces neurotoxicity, contributing to cognitive decline.

Decode the tau protein hyperphosphorylation in cognitive disorders:

$$\text{Tau} + \text{Kinase} \xrightarrow{\text{Hyperphosphorylation}} \text{Neurofibrillary Tangles} \tag{4.18}$$

Hyperphosphorylation of tau proteins leads to the formation of neurofibrillary tangles, impacting cognitive function.

Unravel the disruption of neural oscillations in cognitive decline:

$$\text{Dysregulated Neural Oscillations} = \frac{\text{Normal Neural Synchronization}}{\text{Impaired Neural Synchronization}} \tag{4.19}$$

Cognitive impairments are associated with disrupted neural oscillations and synchronization.

Dive into the impact of cholinergic dysfunction:

$$\text{Acetylcholine} + \text{AChE} \xrightarrow{\text{Deficiency}} \text{Cholinergic Dysfunction} \tag{4.20}$$

Cholinergic dysfunction contributes to cognitive impairments in various disorders.

Conclude with the intricate dance of cognitive impairments and their connection to cognitive waves, where insights guide the understanding of these complex conditions.

4.7 Therapeutic Approaches

Explore therapeutic interventions for neurological disorders and cognitive waves with swift insights:

Illuminate the role of acetylcholinesterase inhibitors:

$$\text{AChE Inhibition} \longrightarrow \text{Increased Acetylcholine} \longrightarrow \text{Improved Cognition} \tag{4.21}$$

Acetylcholinesterase inhibitors enhance acetylcholine levels, improving cognitive function.

Decode the impact of NMDA receptor modulators:

$$\text{NMDA Modulation} \longrightarrow \text{Enhanced Synaptic Plasticity} \longrightarrow \text{Cognitive Improvement} \tag{4.22}$$

Modulating NMDA receptors enhances synaptic plasticity, contributing to cognitive improvement.

Unravel the role of dopamine agonists:

$$\text{Dopamine Agonism} \longrightarrow \text{Improved Dopaminergic Function} \longrightarrow \text{Motor and Cognitive Benefits} \tag{4.23}$$

Dopamine agonists enhance dopaminergic function, providing motor and cognitive benefits.

Dive into the therapeutic potential of GABAergic modulation:

$$\text{GABA Modulation} \longrightarrow \text{Restored Excitation}-\text{Inhibition Balance} \longrightarrow \text{Seizure Control} \tag{4.24}$$

Modulating GABAergic activity restores excitation-inhibition balance, aiding in seizure control.

Conclude with the intricate dance of therapeutic approaches, where insights guide the development of interventions for neurological disorders and cognitive waves.

Chapter 5

Quantitative Analysis Techniques

5.1 Time-Frequency Analysis

Explore the dynamic realm of time-frequency analysis with rapid insights:

Illuminate the essence of Short-Time Fourier Transform (STFT):

$$\text{STFT}(t, f) = \int_{-\infty}^{\infty} x(\tau) \cdot w(t - \tau) \cdot e^{-2\pi i f \tau} \, d\tau$$

STFT unveils the time-varying frequency components of a signal.

Decode the magic of Continuous Wavelet Transform (CWT):

$$\text{CWT}(a, b) = \int_{-\infty}^{\infty} x(t) \cdot \psi^* \left(\frac{t - b}{a} \right) \, dt$$

CWT captures signal variations at different scales and time points.

Unravel the power of Wigner-Ville Distribution (WVD):

$$\text{WVD}(t, f) = \int_{-\infty}^{\infty} x(\tau) \cdot x^*(\tau - t) \cdot e^{-2\pi i f \tau} \, d\tau$$

WVD exposes time-frequency characteristics, overcoming Heisenberg's uncertainty principle.

Dive into the dynamics of Hilbert-Huang Transform (HHT):

$$\text{HHT}(t) = \text{Hilbert Transform[Instantaneous Frequency}(t)]$$

HHT decomposes signals into intrinsic mode functions, offering a detailed time-frequency representation.

Conclude with the dynamic landscape of time-frequency analysis, where these techniques unveil the richness of signal dynamics.

5.2 Spectral Analysis

Delve into the realm of spectral analysis with rapid insights:

Illuminate the Fourier Transform's power:

$$X(f) = \int_{-\infty}^{\infty} x(t) \cdot e^{-2\pi i f t} \, dt$$

Fourier Transform uncovers the frequency components of a signal.

Decode the energy distribution with Power Spectral Density (PSD):

$$\mathrm{PSD}(f) = \lim_{T \to \infty} \frac{1}{T} \cdot |X(f)|^2$$

PSD reveals how signal power distributes across frequencies.

Unravel the coherence between signals with Cross-Spectral Density (CSD):

$$\mathrm{CSD}_{xy}(f) = X_{xy}(f) \cdot X_{yx}^*(f)$$

CSD measures the coherence and phase relationship between two signals.

Dive into the time-varying spectrum with Short-Time Fourier Transform (STFT):

$$\mathrm{STFT}(t, f) = \int_{-\infty}^{\infty} x(\tau) \cdot w(t - \tau) \cdot e^{-2\pi i f \tau} \, d\tau$$

STFT captures spectral variations over time.

Conclude with the dynamic landscape of spectral analysis, where these techniques unveil the frequency intricacies of signals.

5.3 Event-Related Potentials (ERPs)

Dive into the world of Event-Related Potentials (ERPs) with swift insights:

Illuminate the averaging magic:

$$ERP(t) = \frac{1}{N} \sum_{i=1}^{N} x_i(t)$$

ERPs emerge by averaging responses to repeated events, highlighting neural activity.

Decode the P300 wave dynamics:

$$P300(t) = \text{Peak Amplitude at 300 ms}$$

P300 wave signifies cognitive processing and attention.

Unravel the N170 wave mysteries:

$$N170(t) = \text{Negative Peak at 170 ms}$$

N170 reflects face perception and visual processing.

Dive into the realm of mismatch negativity (MMN):

$$MMN(t) = \text{Deviant Stimulus ERP} - \text{Standard Stimulus ERP}$$

MMN captures the brain's response to unexpected stimuli.

Conclude with the dynamic landscape of ERPs, where these potentials unveil the subtleties of cognitive processing.

5.4 Connectivity Measures

Explore the intricacies of connectivity measures with swift insights:

Illuminate the correlation magic:

$$\text{Correlation}(X, Y) = \frac{\text{Covariance}(X, Y)}{\sqrt{\text{Var}(X) \cdot \text{Var}(Y)}}$$

Correlation unveils the linear relationship between two variables.

Decode the power of coherence:

$$\text{Coherence}(f) = \frac{|C_{xy}(f)|^2}{C_{xx}(f) \cdot C_{yy}(f)}$$

Coherence quantifies the degree of synchronization between two signals.

Unravel the Granger causality dynamics:

$$GC(X \rightarrow Y) = \ln\left(\frac{\text{Var}(Y|X)}{\text{Var}(Y|X, \text{Past } Y)}\right)$$

Granger causality measures the predictive power of one time series on another.

Dive into the phase-amplitude coupling wonders:

$$\text{PAC}(f_{\text{phase}}, f_{\text{amplitude}}) = \text{Mean Amplitude at } f_{\text{amplitude}} \text{ in Phase Bins at } f_{\text{phase}}$$

Phase-amplitude coupling reveals interactions between different frequency components.

Conclude with the dynamic landscape of connectivity measures, where these techniques unveil the intricate relationships within neural networks.

5.5 Machine Learning Applications

Embark on the realm of Machine Learning (ML) applications with swift insights:

Illuminate the magic of Support Vector Machines (SVM):

$$\text{SVM Decision Function: } f(x) = \sum_{i=1}^{N} \alpha_i \cdot \text{Kernel}(x_i, x) + b$$

SVM classifies data points by finding the hyperplane with maximum margin.

Decode the elegance of Neural Networks:

$$\text{Feedforward: } y = \sigma(W \cdot x + b)$$

Neural networks learn complex patterns through layers of interconnected neurons.

Unravel the power of Random Forests:

$$\text{Random Forest Prediction: } \bar{y} = \frac{1}{B} \sum_{i=1}^{B} f_i(x)$$

Random Forests aggregate predictions from multiple decision trees, enhancing robustness.

Dive into the wonders of Principal Component Analysis (PCA):

$$\text{PCA Transformation: } \text{PC}_i = \text{Eigenvalue}_i \times \text{Eigenvector}_i$$

PCA extracts principal components, reducing data dimensionality while preserving variance.

Conclude with the dynamic landscape of ML applications, where these techniques unveil patterns, make predictions, and extract insights from complex data.

5.6   Ethical Considerations

Navigate the ethical landscape of quantitative analysis with swift insights:

Illuminate the fairness challenge:

$$\text{Fairness Index} = \frac{\text{True Positive Rate}}{\text{False Positive Rate}}$$

Fairness index measures the balance between true and false positives.

Decode the transparency equation:

$$\text{Transparency} = \frac{\text{Interpretable Model Components}}{\text{Total Model Complexity}}$$

Transparency quantifies the interpretability of models.

Unravel the bias detection mechanism:

$$\text{Bias Detection} = \frac{\text{Prediction Discrepancy}}{\text{Demographic Disparity}}$$

Bias detection assesses disparities in model predictions across different demographics.

Dive into the accountability formula:

$$\text{Accountability} = \frac{\text{Explanatory Power}}{\text{Model Decision Influence}}$$

Accountability gauges how much a model's explanation aligns with its decision-making influence.

Conclude with the dynamic landscape of ethical considerations, where these metrics guide responsible and unbiased quantitative analysis.

5.7   Limitations and Challenges

Navigate the complex terrain of limitations and challenges in quantitative analysis with swift insights:

Illuminate the curse of dimensionality:

$$\text{Curse of Dimensionality} = \frac{\text{Volume in High Dimensions}}{\text{Volume in Low Dimensions}}$$

The curse of dimensionality highlights challenges in sparse data and computational intensity.

Decode the model overfitting menace:

$$\text{Overfitting} = \text{Model Complexity} - \text{Model Generalization}$$

Overfitting occurs when a model captures noise instead of underlying patterns. Unravel the bias-variance tradeoff equation:

$$\text{Bias-Variance Tradeoff} = \text{Model Bias}^2 + \text{Model Variance}$$

The bias-variance tradeoff balances underfitting and overfitting in model performance. Dive into the interpretability dilemma:

$$\text{Interpretability} = \frac{\text{Model Simplicity}}{\text{Model Accuracy}}$$

Achieving interpretability while maintaining accuracy poses a significant challenge.

Conclude with the dynamic landscape of limitations and challenges, where addressing these factors enhances the reliability and effectiveness of quantitative analysis.

Chapter 6

Formulae for Cognitive Enhancement

6.1   Brainwave Entrainment

Unlock the potential of brainwave entrainment with rapid insights:

Illuminate the frequency alignment:

$$\text{Frequency Alignment} = \text{Desired Frequency} - \text{Baseline Frequency}$$

Frequency alignment guides the choice of brainwave frequencies for entrainment.

Decode the binaural beats essence:

$$\text{Binaural Beat Frequency} = \text{Frequency in Left Ear} - \text{Frequency in Right Ear}$$

Binaural beats induce neural synchronization by creating an auditory frequency difference.

Unravel the isochronic tones magic:

$$\text{Isochronic Pulse Frequency} = \text{Regular Pulse Rate}$$

Isochronic tones use a consistent pulse frequency, enhancing brainwave synchronization.

Dive into the entrainment duration formula:

$$\text{Entrainment Duration} = \frac{\text{Total Session Time}}{\text{Number of Entrainment Cycles}}$$

Entrainment duration optimizes the effectiveness of cognitive enhancement sessions.

Conclude with the dynamic landscape of brainwave entrainment, where these formulas guide the pursuit of cognitive enhancement.

6.2 Neurofeedback Techniques

Harness the power of neurofeedback techniques with rapid insights:

Illuminate the Feedback Index (FI):

$$\text{FI} = \frac{\text{Measured Brain Activity}}{\text{Baseline Brain Activity}}$$

The Feedback Index quantifies the deviation of current brain activity from the baseline.

Decode the Reward/Punishment Ratio (RPR):

$$\text{RPR} = \frac{\text{Rewards Earned}}{\text{Punishments Received}}$$

RPR balances reinforcement in neurofeedback, shaping desired brainwave patterns.

Unravel the Self-Regulation Index (SRI):

$$\text{SRI} = \frac{\text{Voluntary Control Duration}}{\text{Total Training Time}}$$

SRI gauges the effectiveness of voluntarily controlling targeted brainwave frequencies.

Dive into the Frequency Band Power Change formula:

$$\text{Power Change} = \frac{\text{Post-Training Power}}{\text{Pre-Training Power}}$$

Power change measures alterations in frequency band power after neurofeedback.

Conclude with the dynamic landscape of neurofeedback techniques, where these formulas guide the path to cognitive enhancement.

6.3 Cognitive Training Programs

Dive into the world of cognitive training programs with swift insights:

Illuminate the Training Intensity equation:

$$\text{Training Intensity} = \frac{\text{Total Cognitive Load}}{\text{Training Duration}}$$

Training intensity balances cognitive load with the duration of the training session.

Decode the Learning Efficiency formula:

$$\text{Learning Efficiency} = \frac{\text{Knowledge Retained}}{\text{Total Learning Time}}$$

Learning efficiency quantifies how effectively knowledge is retained over the learning period.

Unravel the Task-Specific Performance Index (TSPI):

$$\text{TSPI} = \frac{\text{Task Performance Improvement}}{\text{Baseline Task Performance}}$$

TSPI measures the improvement in task-specific performance compared to the baseline.

Dive into the Cognitive Flexibility Score (CFS):

$$\text{CFS} = \frac{\text{Successfully Completed Flexible Tasks}}{\text{Total Flexible Tasks Attempted}}$$

CFS assesses the ability to adapt and switch between different cognitive tasks.

Conclude with the dynamic landscape of cognitive training programs, where these formulas guide the optimization of cognitive enhancement efforts.

6.4 Nutrition and Cognitive Waves

Explore the impact of nutrition on cognitive waves with rapid insights:

Illuminate the Omega-3 Fatty Acids formula:

Omega-3 FAs = (EPA + DHA) / Total Fatty Acids

Omega-3 Fatty Acids, especially EPA and DHA, contribute to cognitive health.

Decode the Antioxidant Power equation:

Antioxidant Power $= \sum (\textit{Concentration of Antioxidant}_i)$

Antioxidants combat oxidative stress, promoting healthy cognitive function.

Unravel the Glucose Metabolism Index (GMI):

GMI = Brain Glucose Utilization / Total Glucose Consumption

GMI assesses the efficiency of glucose utilization in supporting cognitive processes.

Dive into the Neurotransmitter Harmony equation:

Neurotransmitter Harmony = Balanced Ratio of Neurotransmitters / Total Neurotransmitter Concentration

Maintaining a balanced ratio of neurotransmitters supports optimal cognitive function.

Conclude with the dynamic landscape of nutrition and cognitive waves, where these formulas guide the nourishment for cognitive enhancement.

6.5 Mindfulness and Meditation

Immerse in the world of mindfulness and meditation with rapid insights:

Illuminate the Mindfulness Index:

$$\text{Mindfulness Index} = \frac{\text{Present Moment Awareness}}{\text{Total Mental Activity}}$$

The Mindfulness Index gauges the degree of present moment awareness during meditation.

Decode the Meditation Duration formula:

$$\text{Meditation Duration} = \frac{\text{Total Time Spent Meditating}}{\text{Number of Meditation Sessions}}$$

Meditation duration quantifies the average time dedicated to each meditation session.

Unravel the Relaxation Response Index (RRI):

$$\text{RRI} = \frac{\text{Reduction in Physiological Stress Markers}}{\text{Baseline Stress Levels}}$$

RRI measures the effectiveness of meditation in inducing a relaxation response.

Dive into the Mind-Wandering Control equation:

$$\text{Mind-Wandering Control} = \frac{\text{Frequency of Mind-Wandering}}{\text{Conscious Effort to Redirect Attention}}$$

Mind-Wandering Control assesses the ability to redirect attention during mindfulness.

Conclude with the dynamic landscape of mindfulness and meditation, where these formulas guide the path to cognitive enhancement.

6.6 Technological Interventions

Dive into the realm of technological interventions with rapid insights:

Illuminate the Brain-Computer Interface (BCI) Efficiency:

$$\text{BCI Efficiency} = \frac{\text{Accurate Commands Generated}}{\text{Total Commands Attempted}}$$

BCI Efficiency measures the accuracy of generating commands through brain-computer interfaces.

Decode the Virtual Reality (VR) Immersion Index:

$$\text{VR Immersion Index} = \frac{\text{Subjective Immersion Ratings}}{\text{Total VR Exposure Time}}$$

The VR Immersion Index assesses the level of immersion experienced during virtual reality interventions.

Unravel the Transcranial Direct Current Stimulation (tDCS) Effectiveness:

$$\text{tDCS Effectiveness} = \frac{\text{Change in Cognitive Performance}}{\text{Duration of tDCS Application}}$$

tDCS Effectiveness measures the impact of transcranial direct current stimulation on cognitive performance.

Dive into the Electroencephalography (EEG) Signal-to-Noise Ratio (SNR):

$$\text{EEG SNR} = \frac{\text{Amplitude of Desired Signal}}{\text{Amplitude of Background Noise}}$$

EEG SNR quantifies the clarity of desired brain signals against background noise.

Conclude with the dynamic landscape of technological interventions, where these formulas guide the optimization of cognitive enhancement using cutting-edge technologies.

6.7 Holistic Approaches

Embark on the journey of holistic approaches with rapid insights:

Illuminate the Holistic Wellness Index:

$$\text{Holistic Wellness Index} = \frac{\text{Physical Wellness} + \text{Mental Wellness} + \text{Social Wellness} + \text{Environmental Wellness}}{4}$$

The Holistic Wellness Index integrates physical, mental, social, and environmental wellness. Decode the Lifestyle Balance Equation:

$$\text{Lifestyle Balance} = \frac{\text{Work-Life Balance} + \text{Activity Balance} + \text{Restorative Balance}}{3}$$

Lifestyle Balance evaluates the equilibrium between work, activities, and restorative practices. Unravel the Resilience Reservoir Formula:

$$\text{Resilience Reservoir} = \frac{\text{Positive Coping Strategies}}{\text{Total Stressors Encountered}}$$

Resilience Reservoir quantifies the effectiveness of positive coping strategies relative to stressors. Dive into the Mind-Body Harmony Index:

$$\text{Mind-Body Harmony Index} = \frac{\text{Mental Calmness} + \text{Physical Relaxation} + \text{Emotional Equanimity}}{3}$$

Mind-Body Harmony evaluates the synchronization of mental calmness, physical relaxation, and emotional equanimity.

Conclude with the dynamic landscape of holistic approaches, where these formulas guide the pursuit of cognitive enhancement through a comprehensive wellness perspective.

Chapter 7

Applications in Various Fields

7.1 Neuromarketing

Explore the realm of neuromarketing with rapid insights:

Illuminate the Neuroengagement Index:

$$\text{Neuroengagement Index} = \frac{\text{Neurological Activation in Response}}{\text{Total Attention Metrics}}$$

The Neuroengagement Index gauges the level of neurological activation in response to marketing stimuli.

Decode the Emotional Resonance Quotient (ERQ):

$$\text{ERQ} = \frac{\text{Emotional Impact}}{\text{Cognitive Processing}}$$

ERQ measures the balance between emotional impact and cognitive processing in marketing.

Unravel the Brand Perception Equation:

$$\text{Brand Perception} = \frac{\text{Positive Neurological Associations}}{\text{Negative Neurological Associations}}$$

Brand Perception assesses the balance of positive and negative neurological associations with a brand.

Dive into the Purchase Intent Probability (PIP):

$$\text{PIP} = \frac{\text{Neurological Activation in Decision-Making Areas}}{\text{Total Decision-Making Metrics}}$$

PIP estimates the probability of purchase intent based on neurological activation in decision-making areas.

Conclude with the dynamic landscape of neuromarketing, where these formulas guide the understanding and optimization of consumer engagement.

7.2   Education and Learning

Delve into the applications of neuroscience in education and learning with rapid insights:

Illuminate the Learning Efficiency Formula:

$$\text{Learning Efficiency} = \frac{\text{Knowledge Retained}}{\text{Total Learning Time}}$$

Learning Efficiency quantifies how effectively knowledge is retained over the learning period.

Decode the Cognitive Load Index (CLI):

$$\text{CLI} = \frac{\text{Intrinsic Cognitive Load} + \text{Extraneous Cognitive Load}}{\text{Germane Cognitive Load}}$$

CLI evaluates the balance between intrinsic, extraneous, and germane cognitive loads during learning.

Unravel the Memory Consolidation Score (MCS):

$$\text{MCS} = \frac{\text{Consolidated Memory Strength}}{\text{Initial Memory Strength}}$$

MCS measures the strength of memory consolidation compared to initial memory strength.

Dive into the Active Engagement Quotient (AEQ):

$$\text{AEQ} = \frac{\text{Active Participation Metrics}}{\text{Total Learning Interaction Metrics}}$$

AEQ assesses the level of active engagement and participation in the learning process.

Conclude with the dynamic landscape of neuroscience in education, where these formulas guide the enhancement of learning outcomes.

7.3   Sports Performance

Uncover the applications of neuroscience in sports performance with rapid insights:

Illuminate the Performance Enhancement Index:

$$\text{Performance Enhancement Index} = \frac{\text{Neurological Activation during Performance}}{\text{Baseline Neurological Activation}}$$

The Performance Enhancement Index quantifies the improvement in neurological activation during sports performance.

Decode the Reaction Time Optimization Formula:

$$\text{Reaction Time Optimization} = \frac{\text{Preparation Time}}{\text{Execution Time}}$$

Reaction Time Optimization assesses the efficiency in reducing the preparation and execution time during sports actions.

Unravel the Motor Skill Consolidation Score (MSCS):

$$\text{MSCS} = \frac{\text{Consolidated Motor Skill Strength}}{\text{Initial Motor Skill Strength}}$$

MSCS measures the strength of motor skill consolidation compared to initial motor skill strength.

Dive into the Focus and Precision Quotient (FPQ):

$$\text{FPQ} = \frac{\text{Focused Attention Metrics}}{\text{Precision in Performance Metrics}}$$

FPQ evaluates the balance between focused attention and precision in sports performance.

Conclude with the dynamic landscape of neuroscience in sports, where these formulas guide the optimization of athletic capabilities.

7.4 Workplace Productivity

Explore the applications of neuroscience in workplace productivity with rapid insights:

Illuminate the Focus and Efficiency Equation:

$$\text{Focus and Efficiency} = \frac{\text{Focused Work Time}}{\text{Total Work Time}}$$

Focus and Efficiency quantify the proportion of time spent on focused work compared to the total work time.

Decode the Cognitive Fatigue Index (CFI):

$$\text{CFI} = \frac{\text{Mental Alertness}}{\text{Perceived Mental Fatigue}}$$

CFI measures the balance between mental alertness and perceived mental fatigue in the workplace.

Unravel the Collaboration Effectiveness Score (CES):

$$\text{CES} = \frac{\text{Positive Collaborative Outcomes}}{\text{Total Collaborative Interactions}}$$

CES assesses the effectiveness of collaboration through positive outcomes relative to total collaborative interactions.

Dive into the Stress Resilience Quotient (SRQ):

$$\text{SRQ} = \frac{\text{Stress Coping Strategies}}{\text{Total Stressors Encountered}}$$

SRQ quantifies the effectiveness of stress coping strategies in the workplace.

Conclude with the dynamic landscape of neuroscience in enhancing workplace productivity, where these formulas guide the optimization of cognitive performance in professional settings.

7.5   Artificial Intelligence

Navigate the applications of neuroscience in artificial intelligence with rapid insights:

Illuminate the Learning Algorithm Efficiency:

$$\text{Learning Algorithm Efficiency} = \frac{\text{Algorithm Accuracy}}{\text{Computational Resources Used}}$$

Learning Algorithm Efficiency gauges the accuracy of AI algorithms relative to the computational resources utilized.

Decode the Neural Network Adaptability Index:

$$\text{Neural Network Adaptability Index} = \frac{\text{Adaptation Speed}}{\text{Learning Data Variability}}$$

The Neural Network Adaptability Index assesses the speed of adaptation and learning variability in neural networks.

Unravel the Decision-Making Precision Quotient (DMPQ):

$$DMPQ = \frac{\text{Precision in Decision Outputs}}{\text{Total Decision Outputs}}$$

DMPQ quantifies the precision in decision outputs generated by artificial intelligence.

Dive into the Creativity Generation Score (CGS):

$$CGS = \frac{\text{Novel Creative Outputs}}{\text{Total Outputs Generated}}$$

CGS evaluates the capacity of AI to generate novel and creative outputs.

Conclude with the dynamic landscape of neuroscience in shaping artificial intelligence, where these formulas guide the development and optimization of intelligent systems.

7.6 Virtual Reality

Immerse into the applications of neuroscience in virtual reality with rapid insights:

Illuminate the Immersion Enhancement Index:

$$\text{Immersion Enhancement Index} = \frac{\text{Subjective Immersion Ratings}}{\text{Total VR Exposure Time}}$$

The Immersion Enhancement Index quantifies the level of immersion experienced by users during virtual reality experiences.

Decode the Motion Sickness Mitigation Formula:

$$\text{Motion Sickness Mitigation} = \frac{\text{Physiological Adaptation Rate}}{\text{Intensity of VR Motion}}$$

Motion Sickness Mitigation assesses the effectiveness of physiological adaptation in reducing the impact of VR motion sickness.

Unravel the Spatial Navigation Efficiency Score (SNES):

$$SNES = \frac{\text{Accuracy in Spatial Navigation}}{\text{Total Navigation Time}}$$

SNES measures the efficiency of spatial navigation in virtual reality environments.

Dive into the Presence and Engagement Quotient (PEQ):

$$PEQ = \frac{\text{Sense of Presence}}{\text{Level of Engagement}}$$

PEQ evaluates the balance between the sense of presence and the level of engagement in virtual reality.

Conclude with the dynamic landscape of neuroscience in enhancing virtual reality experiences, where these formulas guide the development and optimization of immersive environments.

7.7 Human-Computer Interaction

Explore the applications of neuroscience in human-computer interaction with rapid insights:

Illuminate the Interface Usability Index:

$$\text{Interface Usability Index} = \frac{\text{User Satisfaction}}{\text{Task Completion Time}}$$

The Interface Usability Index gauges user satisfaction relative to the time taken to complete tasks.

Decode the Attention and Interface Engagement Quotient (AIEQ):

$$\text{AIEQ} = \frac{\text{Attention Allocation}}{\text{Level of Interface Engagement}}$$

AIEQ assesses the balance between attention allocation and the level of engagement with computer interfaces.

Unravel the Interaction Efficiency Score (IES):

$$\text{IES} = \frac{\text{Efficiency in Interaction}}{\text{Cognitive Effort Expended}}$$

IES measures the efficiency of user interaction with computer interfaces relative to cognitive effort.

Dive into the Error Recovery Resilience Formula:

$$\text{Error Recovery Resilience} = \frac{\text{Successful Error Recoveries}}{\text{Total Errors Encountered}}$$

Error Recovery Resilience quantifies the success rate of recovering from errors during human-computer interaction.

Conclude with the dynamic landscape of neuroscience in optimizing human-computer interaction, where these formulas guide the design and usability of digital interfaces.

Chapter 8

Future Trends and Emerging Technologies

8.1 Advancements in EEG Technology

Dive into the future of EEG technology with rapid insights:

Illuminate the Spatial Resolution Enhancement Formula:

$$\text{Spatial Resolution Enhancement} = \frac{\text{Number of Electrodes}}{\text{Inter-Electrode Distance}}$$

Spatial Resolution Enhancement quantifies the improvement in spatial resolution based on the number of electrodes and their inter-electrode distance.

Decode the Temporal Precision Boost Index:

$$\text{Temporal Precision Boost Index} = \frac{\text{Temporal Sampling Rate}}{\text{Signal-to-Noise Ratio}}$$

Temporal Precision Boost Index assesses the improvement in temporal precision through a higher sampling rate relative to the signal-to-noise ratio.

Unravel the Connectivity Mapping Accuracy Score (CMAS):

$$\text{CMAS} = \frac{\text{Accuracy in Connectivity Mapping}}{\text{Computational Processing Time}}$$

CMAS measures the accuracy of connectivity mapping in EEG with consideration for computational processing time.

Dive into the Wireless EEG Data Transmission Efficiency:

$$\text{Wireless EEG Data Transmission Efficiency} = \frac{\text{Data Transfer Rate}}{\text{Energy Consumption}}$$

Wireless EEG Data Transmission Efficiency evaluates the efficiency of transmitting EEG data wirelessly in terms of data transfer rate and energy consumption.

Conclude with the dynamic landscape of advancements in EEG technology, where these formulas guide the future developments and optimization of electroencephalography.

8.2 Neuropharmacology

Explore the future of neuropharmacology with rapid insights:

Illuminate the Neurotransmitter Modulation Quotient:

$$\text{Neurotransmitter Modulation Quotient} = \frac{\text{Modulation Effect on Neurotransmitter Release}}{\text{Drug Dosage}}$$

The Neurotransmitter Modulation Quotient quantifies the modulation effect on neurotransmitter release relative to the dosage of a neuropharmacological drug.

Decode the Receptor Sensitivity Optimization Index:

$$\text{Receptor Sensitivity Optimization Index} = \frac{\text{Receptor Sensitivity Enhancement}}{\text{Drug Half-Life}}$$

Receptor Sensitivity Optimization Index assesses the enhancement in receptor sensitivity over the drug's half-life.

Unravel the Neuroprotective Efficacy Score (NES):

$$\text{NES} = \frac{\text{Neuroprotective Effects}}{\text{Adverse Side Effects}}$$

NES measures the neuroprotective efficacy of a drug relative to its adverse side effects.

Dive into the Blood-Brain Barrier Permeability Formula:

$$\text{Blood-Brain Barrier Permeability} = \frac{\text{Drug Concentration in Brain Tissue}}{\text{Drug Concentration in Blood Plasma}}$$

Blood-Brain Barrier Permeability assesses the ability of a drug to permeate the blood-brain barrier.

Conclude with the dynamic landscape of neuropharmacology, where these formulas guide the future development and optimization of pharmacological interventions.

8.3 Brain-Computer Interfaces

Embark on the future of Brain-Computer Interfaces (BCIs) with rapid insights:

Illuminate the Information Transfer Rate Amplification:

$$\text{Information Transfer Rate Amplification} = \frac{\text{Bit Rate of Brain Signals}}{\text{Signal-to-Noise Ratio}}$$

Information Transfer Rate Amplification quantifies the amplification in information transfer rate based on the bit rate of brain signals and signal-to-noise ratio.

Decode the Neural Command Precision Quotient (NCPQ):

$$\text{NCPQ} = \frac{\text{Precision in Neural Commands}}{\text{Time Interval between Commands}}$$

NCPQ assesses the precision of neural commands relative to the time interval between consecutive commands.

Unravel the Cortical Mapping Resolution Index:

$$\text{Cortical Mapping Resolution Index} = \frac{\text{Resolution of Cortical Mapping}}{\text{Computational Processing Time}}$$

Cortical Mapping Resolution Index measures the resolution of cortical mapping in BCIs with consideration for computational processing time.

Dive into the Biocompatibility and Longevity Formula:

$$\text{Biocompatibility and Longevity} = \frac{\text{Biocompatibility Score}}{\text{Device Lifespan}}$$

Biocompatibility and Longevity assess the biocompatibility of BCIs and their overall lifespan.

Conclude with the dynamic landscape of Brain-Computer Interfaces, where these formulas guide the future advancements and optimization of neural interfaces.

8.4   Precision Medicine

Delve into the future of precision medicine with rapid insights:

Illuminate the Genetic Profiling Accuracy Score:

$$\text{Genetic Profiling Accuracy Score} = \frac{\text{Accuracy in Identifying Genetic Variants}}{\text{Computational Processing Time}}$$

Genetic Profiling Accuracy Score quantifies the accuracy in identifying genetic variants with consideration for computational processing time.

Decode the Personalized Treatment Response Index:

$$\text{Personalized Treatment Response Index} = \frac{\text{Effectiveness of Treatment}}{\text{Patient-Specific Factors}}$$

Personalized Treatment Response Index assesses the effectiveness of treatment considering patient-specific factors.

Unravel the Biomarker Discovery Efficiency:

$$\text{Biomarker Discovery Efficiency} = \frac{\text{Number of Validated Biomarkers}}{\text{Research and Development Investment}}$$

Biomarker Discovery Efficiency measures the efficiency in discovering validated biomarkers relative to the investment in research and development.

Dive into the Therapeutic Dose Optimization Formula:

$$\text{Therapeutic Dose Optimization} = \frac{\text{Optimal Therapeutic Dose}}{\text{Individual Patient Characteristics}}$$

Therapeutic Dose Optimization assesses the optimization of therapeutic doses considering individual patient characteristics.

Conclude with the dynamic landscape of precision medicine, where these formulas guide the future developments and optimization of personalized healthcare.

8.5   Big Data and Analytics

Dive into the future of Big Data and Analytics with rapid insights:

Illuminate the Data Integration Efficiency Quotient:

$$\text{Data Integration Efficiency Quotient} = \frac{\text{Integration Accuracy}}{\text{Processing Time}}$$

Data Integration Efficiency Quotient quantifies the accuracy of integrating diverse data sources relative to the processing time.

Decode the Predictive Modeling Accuracy Score:

$$\text{Predictive Modeling Accuracy Score} = \frac{\text{Model Accuracy}}{\text{Volume of Data}}$$

Predictive Modeling Accuracy Score assesses the accuracy of predictive models in relation to the volume of data processed.

Unravel the Anomaly Detection Sensitivity Index:

$$\text{Anomaly Detection Sensitivity Index} = \frac{\text{Sensitivity in Detecting Anomalies}}{\text{False Positive Rate}}$$

Anomaly Detection Sensitivity Index measures the sensitivity in detecting anomalies while considering the false positive rate.

Dive into the Computational Resource Utilization Efficiency:

$$\text{Computational Resource Utilization Efficiency} = \frac{\text{Analytical Output}}{\text{Computational Resources Consumed}}$$

Computational Resource Utilization Efficiency assesses the efficiency of generating analytical output relative to the computational resources consumed.

Conclude with the dynamic landscape of Big Data and Analytics, where these formulas guide the future advancements and optimization of data-driven decision-making.

8.6 Global Collaborations

Explore the future of global collaborations in scientific research with rapid insights:

Illuminate the Collaborative Impact Index:

$$\text{Collaborative Impact Index} = \frac{\text{Research Impact}}{\text{Number of Collaborators}}$$

Collaborative Impact Index quantifies the research impact achieved through global collaborations relative to the number of collaborators involved.

Decode the Knowledge Exchange Efficiency Quotient:

$$\text{Knowledge Exchange Efficiency Quotient} = \frac{\text{Effective Knowledge Exchange}}{\text{Communication Overhead}}$$

Knowledge Exchange Efficiency Quotient assesses the efficiency of knowledge exchange during global collaborations considering communication overhead.

Unravel the Cross-Disciplinary Synergy Score (CDSS):

$$\text{CDSS} = \frac{\text{Synergy in Cross-Disciplinary Collaborations}}{\text{Disciplinary Diversity Index}}$$

CDSS measures the synergy achieved in cross-disciplinary collaborations relative to the diversity of disciplines involved.

Dive into the Global Research Productivity Formula:

$$\text{Global Research Productivity} = \frac{\text{Number of Collaborative Publications}}{\text{Total Research Investment}}$$

Global Research Productivity assesses the research output achieved through global collaborations relative to the total research investment.

Conclude with the dynamic landscape of global collaborations, where these formulas guide the future of collaborative research endeavors.

8.7 Societal Impacts and Considerations

Delve into the future societal impacts and considerations of emerging technologies with rapid insights:

Illuminate the Ethical AI Adoption Index:

$$\text{Ethical AI Adoption Index} = \frac{\text{Organizational Adoption of Ethical AI Practices}}{\text{Algorithmic Bias Mitigation}}$$

Ethical AI Adoption Index quantifies the level of organizational adoption of ethical AI practices relative to the effectiveness of algorithmic bias mitigation.

Decode the Digital Inclusion Progress Score:

$$\text{Digital Inclusion Progress Score} = \frac{\text{Progress in Digital Inclusion Initiatives}}{\text{Socioeconomic Inequality Index}}$$

Digital Inclusion Progress Score assesses the progress in digital inclusion initiatives considering the socioeconomic inequality index.

Unravel the Technology Accessibility Quotient:

$$\text{Technology Accessibility Quotient} = \frac{\text{Accessibility of Technologies}}{\text{User Adoption Rate}}$$

Technology Accessibility Quotient measures the accessibility of technologies relative to the user adoption rate.

Dive into the Environmental Sustainability Impact Formula:

$$\text{Environmental Sustainability Impact} = \frac{\text{Technology Adoption Impact on Environment}}{\text{Sustainable Practices Integration}}$$

Environmental Sustainability Impact assesses the impact of technology adoption on the environment considering the integration of sustainable practices.

Conclude with the dynamic landscape of societal impacts and considerations, where these formulas guide the responsible development and deployment of emerging technologies.

Chapter 9

Case Studies

9.1   Successful Cognitive Enhancement

Explore case studies showcasing successful cognitive enhancement with rapid insights:

Illuminate the Cognitive Performance Index (CPI):

$$\text{CPI} = \frac{\text{Post-Enhancement Cognitive Performance}}{\text{Pre-Enhancement Cognitive Performance}}$$

Cognitive Performance Index quantifies the improvement in cognitive performance post-enhancement relative to the baseline performance.

Decode the Learning Acceleration Coefficient:

$$\text{Learning Acceleration Coefficient} = \frac{\text{Rate of Learning Acceleration}}{\text{Enhancement Intervention Duration}}$$

Learning Acceleration Coefficient assesses the rate of learning acceleration achieved through cognitive enhancement interventions over the intervention duration.

Unravel the Neuroplasticity Resilience Score:

$$\text{Neuroplasticity Resilience Score} = \frac{\text{Resilience of Neuroplasticity Mechanisms}}{\text{Cognitive Fatigue Recovery Time}}$$

Neuroplasticity Resilience Score measures the resilience of neuroplasticity mechanisms relative to the recovery time from cognitive fatigue.

Dive into the Memory Retention Sustainability Index:

$$\text{Memory Retention Sustainability Index} = \frac{\text{Sustainability of Memory Retention}}{\text{Intervention Adherence Rate}}$$

Memory Retention Sustainability Index assesses the sustainability of memory retention achieved through cognitive enhancement interventions considering the adherence rate.

Conclude with these case studies, illustrating the successful application of cognitive enhancement interventions and the corresponding quantitative metrics.

9.2 Rehabilitation Success Stories

Explore rehabilitation success stories with rapid insights:

Illuminate the Functional Recovery Index (FRI):

$$\text{FRI} = \frac{\text{Post-Rehabilitation Functional Level}}{\text{Pre-Rehabilitation Functional Level}}$$

Functional Recovery Index quantifies the improvement in functional level post-rehabilitation relative to the baseline functional level.

Decode the Motor Skill Restoration Quotient:

$$\text{Motor Skill Restoration Quotient} = \frac{\text{Restoration in Motor Skills}}{\text{Rehabilitation Duration}}$$

Motor Skill Restoration Quotient assesses the restoration in motor skills achieved through rehabilitation interventions over the rehabilitation duration.

Unravel the Neuromuscular Adaptation Efficiency:

$$\text{Neuromuscular Adaptation Efficiency} = \frac{\text{Efficiency in Neuromuscular Adaptation}}{\text{Rehabilitation Adherence Rate}}$$

Neuromuscular Adaptation Efficiency measures the efficiency in neuromuscular adaptation achieved through rehabilitation considering the adherence rate.

Dive into the Pain Management Success Score:

$$\text{Pain Management Success Score} = \frac{\text{Success in Pain Management}}{\text{Patient Reported Pain Severity Reduction}}$$

Pain Management Success Score assesses the success in pain management relative to the reduction in patient-reported pain severity.

Conclude with these rehabilitation success stories, highlighting the positive outcomes and quantitative metrics of the rehabilitation interventions.

9.3 Innovative Research Projects

Explore case studies of innovative research projects with rapid insights:

Illuminate the Research Impact Quotient:

$$\text{Research Impact Quotient} = \frac{\text{Project Impact}}{\text{Investment and Resource Utilization}}$$

Research Impact Quotient quantifies the impact of the research project relative to the investment and resources utilized.

Decode the Scientific Collaboration Effectiveness Index:

$$\text{Scientific Collaboration Effectiveness Index} = \frac{\text{Collaboration Productivity}}{\text{Communication Overhead}}$$

Scientific Collaboration Effectiveness Index assesses the productivity of scientific collaborations considering the communication overhead.

Unravel the Technological Innovation Efficiency:

$$\text{Technological Innovation Efficiency} = \frac{\text{Innovation Output}}{\text{Research and Development Investment}}$$

Technological Innovation Efficiency measures the efficiency in technological innovation relative to the investment in research and development.

Dive into the Cross-Disciplinary Integration Score:

$$\text{Cross-Disciplinary Integration Score} = \frac{\text{Integration of Disciplines}}{\text{Project Success Rate}}$$

Cross-Disciplinary Integration Score quantifies the integration of disciplines in the research project relative to the project success rate.

Conclude with these case studies, showcasing the success and impact of innovative research projects, supported by quantitative metrics.

9.4   Cross-Disciplinary Applications

Explore case studies of cross-disciplinary applications with rapid insights:

Illuminate the Interdisciplinary Impact Quotient:

$$\text{Interdisciplinary Impact Quotient} = \frac{\text{Impact of Interdisciplinary Integration}}{\text{Disciplinary Autonomy}}$$

Interdisciplinary Impact Quotient quantifies the impact achieved through interdisciplinary integration relative to disciplinary autonomy.

Decode the Knowledge Transfer Velocity:

$$\text{Knowledge Transfer Velocity} = \frac{\text{Velocity of Knowledge Transfer}}{\text{Communication Latency}}$$

Knowledge Transfer Velocity assesses the speed of knowledge transfer in cross-disciplinary applications considering communication latency.

Unravel the Innovation Synergy Score:

$$\text{Innovation Synergy Score} = \frac{\text{Synergy in Innovation}}{\text{Cross-Disciplinary Collaboration Density}}$$

Innovation Synergy Score measures the synergy achieved in innovation through cross-disciplinary collaboration relative to collaboration density.

Dive into the Impactful Collaboration Formula:

$$\text{Impactful Collaboration} = \frac{\text{Project Impact}}{\text{Collaborative Effort Contribution}}$$

Impactful Collaboration assesses the impact of collaborative efforts in cross-disciplinary applications relative to individual contributions.

Conclude with these case studies, showcasing the successful integration of diverse disciplines and the quantitative metrics supporting their impact.

9.5   Challenges Overcome

Explore case studies of overcoming challenges with rapid insights:

Illuminate the Resilience Quotient:

$$\text{Resilience Quotient} = \frac{\text{Level of Challenge Overcome}}{\text{Resource Utilization}}$$

Resilience Quotient quantifies the level of challenge overcome relative to the resources utilized.

Decode the Adaptive Innovation Index:

$$\text{Adaptive Innovation Index} = \frac{\text{Innovation Rate}}{\text{Adaptation Effort}}$$

Adaptive Innovation Index assesses the rate of innovation achieved relative to the effort invested in adaptation.

Unravel the Collaboration Effectiveness Ratio:

$$\text{Collaboration Effectiveness Ratio} = \frac{\text{Effectiveness of Collaboration}}{\text{Collaboration Complexity}}$$

Collaboration Effectiveness Ratio measures the effectiveness of collaboration in overcoming challenges considering the complexity of collaboration.

Dive into the Persistence Success Score:

$$\text{Persistence Success Score} = \frac{\text{Success Achieved}}{\text{Persistence Duration}}$$

Persistence Success Score assesses the success achieved relative to the duration of persistence in overcoming challenges.

Conclude with these case studies, showcasing resilience, innovation, collaboration, and persistence in overcoming challenges, supported by quantitative metrics.

9.6 Unanswered Questions

Explore case studies of unanswered questions with rapid insights:

Illuminate the Inquiry Complexity Index:

$$\text{Inquiry Complexity Index} = \frac{\text{Complexity of Unanswered Questions}}{\text{Research Effort Invested}}$$

Inquiry Complexity Index quantifies the complexity of unanswered questions relative to the research effort invested.

Decode the Knowledge Gap Magnitude:

$$\text{Knowledge Gap Magnitude} = \frac{\text{Magnitude of Unanswered Knowledge Gaps}}{\text{Information Accessibility}}$$

Knowledge Gap Magnitude assesses the magnitude of unanswered knowledge gaps relative to the accessibility of information.

Unravel the Question Relevance Quotient:

$$\text{Question Relevance Quotient} = \frac{\text{Relevance of Unanswered Questions}}{\text{Research Impact Potential}}$$

Question Relevance Quotient measures the relevance of unanswered questions relative to their potential impact on research.

Dive into the Curiosity Unexplored Score:

$$\text{Curiosity Unexplored Score} = \frac{\text{Unexplored Curiosity}}{\text{Research Exploration Efficiency}}$$

Curiosity Unexplored Score assesses the unexplored aspects of curiosity relative to the efficiency of research exploration.

Conclude with these case studies, highlighting the complexity, magnitude, relevance, and unexplored curiosity of unanswered questions, supported by quantitative metrics.

9.7   Lessons Learned

Explore case studies of lessons learned with rapid insights:

Illuminate the Wisdom Accumulation Index:

$$\text{Wisdom Accumulation Index} = \frac{\text{Accumulated Wisdom}}{\text{Experience Duration}}$$

Wisdom Accumulation Index quantifies the accumulated wisdom relative to the duration of experience.

Decode the Adaptability Quotient:

$$\text{Adaptability Quotient} = \frac{\text{Rate of Adaptation}}{\text{Lesson Implementation Efficiency}}$$

Adaptability Quotient assesses the rate of adaptation achieved relative to the efficiency of implementing lessons learned.

Unravel the Decision-Making Confidence Score:

$$\text{Decision-Making Confidence Score} = \frac{\text{Confidence in Decision-Making}}{\text{Lesson Integration Depth}}$$

Decision-Making Confidence Score measures the confidence in decision-making relative to the depth of integration of lessons learned.

Dive into the Innovation Resilience Factor:

$$\text{Innovation Resilience Factor} = \frac{\text{Resilience in Innovation}}{\text{Lesson Implementation Success}}$$

Innovation Resilience Factor assesses the resilience achieved in innovation relative to the success of implementing lessons learned.

Conclude with these case studies, showcasing the accumulation of wisdom, adaptability, decision-making confidence, and innovation resilience through lessons learned, supported by quantitative metrics.

Chapter 10

Conclusion

10.1 Summary of Key Findings

Summarize the key findings with rapid insights:

Illuminate the Comprehensive Impact Index:

$$\text{Comprehensive Impact Index} = \frac{\text{Total Impact}}{\text{Holistic Assessment Factors}}$$

Comprehensive Impact Index provides a holistic measure of the total impact considering various assessment factors.

Decode the Knowledge Integration Coefficient:

$$\text{Knowledge Integration Coefficient} = \frac{\text{Integration of Knowledge Domains}}{\text{Interdisciplinary Collaboration Strength}}$$

Knowledge Integration Coefficient assesses the integration of knowledge domains relative to the strength of interdisciplinary collaboration.

Unravel the Innovation Synergy Quotient:

$$\text{Innovation Synergy Quotient} = \frac{\text{Synergy in Innovation Strategies}}{\text{Collaboration Effectiveness}}$$

Innovation Synergy Quotient measures the synergy achieved in innovation strategies relative to collaboration effectiveness.

Dive into the Transformational Impact Score:

$$\text{Transformational Impact Score} = \frac{\text{Impact on Cognitive Sciences}}{\text{Societal and Technological Transformations}}$$

Transformational Impact Score assesses the impact on cognitive sciences relative to societal and technological transformations.

Conclude with a comprehensive summary of these key findings, showcasing the overall impact, knowledge integration, innovation synergy, and transformational impact of cognitive wave research, supported by quantitative metrics.

Chapter 11

Conclusion

11.1　Implications for the Future

Explore the implications for the future with rapid insights:

Illuminate the Cognitive Revolution Quotient:

$$\text{Cognitive Revolution Quotient} = \frac{\text{Revolutionary Impact}}{\text{Future Relevance}}$$

Cognitive Revolution Quotient quantifies the revolutionary impact relative to the future relevance of cognitive wave research.

Decode the Ethical Advancement Index:

$$\text{Ethical Advancement Index} = \frac{\text{Advancement in Ethical Considerations}}{\text{Technological Integration Ethicality}}$$

Ethical Advancement Index assesses the advancement in ethical considerations relative to the ethicality of integrating technologies in the future.

Unravel the Societal Harmony Coefficient:

$$\text{Societal Harmony Coefficient} = \frac{\text{Harmony in Societal Integration}}{\text{Acceptance of Cognitive Technologies}}$$

Societal Harmony Coefficient measures the harmony achieved in societal integration relative to the acceptance of cognitive technologies.

Dive into the Cognitive Resilience Score:

$$\text{Cognitive Resilience Score} = \frac{\text{Resilience in Cognitive Systems}}{\text{Adaptability to Emerging Challenges}}$$

Cognitive Resilience Score assesses the resilience in cognitive systems relative to adaptability to emerging challenges.

Conclude with a forward-looking perspective, exploring the cognitive revolution, ethical advancement, societal harmony, and cognitive resilience implications for the future, supported by quantitative metrics.

11.2   Closing Thoughts

Conclude with closing thoughts and reflections:

Illuminate the Visionary Insight Index:

$$\text{Visionary Insight Index} = \frac{\text{Insightfulness in Closing Thoughts}}{\text{Inspiration Impact}}$$

Visionary Insight Index quantifies the insightful nature of closing thoughts relative to their impact on inspiration.

Decode the Reflective Wisdom Quotient:

$$\text{Reflective Wisdom Quotient} = \frac{\text{Wisdom in Reflection}}{\text{Emotional Resonance}}$$

Reflective Wisdom Quotient assesses the wisdom conveyed in reflections relative to their emotional resonance.

Unravel the Inspirational Depth Score:

$$\text{Inspirational Depth Score} = \frac{\text{Depth of Inspiration}}{\text{Resonance with Key Themes}}$$

Inspirational Depth Score measures the depth of inspiration conveyed relative to the resonance with key themes.

Dive into the Timeless Impact Coefficient:

$$\text{Timeless Impact Coefficient} = \frac{\text{Timeless Relevance}}{\text{Memorability Factor}}$$

Timeless Impact Coefficient assesses the timeless relevance of closing thoughts relative to their memorability factor.

Conclude with these closing thoughts, emphasizing visionary insights, reflective wisdom, inspirational depth, and timeless impact, supported by quantitative metrics.